THE
ALKALINE LIFE

LOOK MARVELOUS AND LOSE WEIGHT NATURALLY

Flip Mcgyver

Table of Contents

INTRODUCTION... 1

CHAPTER 1 4

WHAT IS AN ALKALINE LIFESTYLE?

CHAPTER 2 7

WHAT IS THE ACID ALKALINE DIET?

CHAPTER 3 9

PRINCIPLES OF THE ALKALINE DIET

CHAPTER 4 12

THE EFFECTS OF ACIDITY AND ALKALINITY ON THE BODY

CHAPTER 5 14

REASONS TO GO ALKALINE AND AVOID ACIDS

CHAPTER 6 19

GETTING STARTED WITH THE ALKALINE DIET

CHAPTER 7 24

ALKALINE DIET AND ITS HEALTH BENEFITS

CHAPTER 8 28

GUIDELINES TO MAINTAINING A HEALTHY ALKALINE BALANCE

CHAPTER 9 32

HOW TO IMPROVE THE ALKALINITY OF YOUR BODY AND BE
HEALTHIER

CHAPTER 10 34

USING A LIST OF PH OF FOODS FOR HEALTH, ENERGY AND WEIGHT

CHAPTER 11 .... **37**

ACID-ALKALINE FOODS

CHAPTER 12 .... **41**

TOP 10 MOST ALKALINE FOODS FOR YOUR DIET

CHAPTER 13 .... **45**

ALKALIZING OUR BODIES WITH FRESH FRUITS AND VEGETABLES

CHAPTER 14 .... **49**

EXAMINING GOOD FOOD WITH ALKALINE DIET CHAR ....

CHAPTER 15 .... **52**

TOP WAYS TO ACHIEVE ALKALINE PH IN YOUR BODY

CHAPTER 16 .... **54**

TIPS TO MAKE THE ALKALINE DIET SUCCESSFUL FOR YOU

CHAPTER 17 .... **56**

GETTING ALKALINE WITH COOL SHORTCUTS

CHAPTER 18 .... **59**

ALKALINITY AS THE SWEET LIFE

CONCLUSION **62**

Introduction

THANK YOU for purchasing your copy of THE ALKALINE LIFE & allowing me to enlighten you about the benefits of having a alkaline body. I look forward to teaching the world about all the health benefits this diet consists of so everyone on the planet can live there best life..... GOD BLESS & ENJOY!

"THE ALKALINE LIFE".

Going back to our more ancient past, man relied on wild vegetation and wild animals for food. When agriculture was discovered, we now had other means of sustaining ourselves aside from hunting and foraging.

After the development of stone tools, grains could easily be consumed. When rolling and sifting devices were developed, refined grains entered the picture. After domesticating animals for livestock, meat and dairy products were in abundance.

When we discovered salt mines, salt for flavoring became popular. As the industrial revolution took place, sugar was in demand. Today, we find more ways to produce more food items that would surely overwhelm our ancestors.

However, the advancements in manufacturing, processing, and mass production took its toll on our health. The very food that was supposedly meant to feed and nourish us is the cause of our own demise.

Whenever we digest food, it is either causes alkalinity or acidity. The two should share a certain balance. Sadly, the modern food that we eat is more acidic than it is alkaline.

Our blood must be slightly alkaline at all times. Whenever it shifts to acidic, this is when we experience a variety of health problems. These health problems are hypertension, heart problems, obesity, diabetes, and cancer. Every disease known to mankind is caused by acidity.

Today, there are many reasons why individuals indulge in the alkaline diet. Some use it as a preventive measure against diseases. Some use it as a cure for their condition. Some simply use it to lose the unwanted pounds. There is one thing that they have in common, and that is to get healthy.

This diet can do a lot for you. It can increase your energy levels; it prevents the production of mucus; it prevents and cures nasal congestion; it prevents and cures common illnesses such as influenza; it alleviates sensations like anxiety and irritability; it is a cure for and prevents chronic headaches, it prevents the recurrence of cancer, and it prevents the disease from ever happening.

The medical world is still divided when it comes to validating the diet's effectiveness. However, they cannot deny the hazards caused by western influenced diets. These diets are mostly acid forming foods, which is the reason why more and more people from western influenced countries are experiencing health risks.

To prevent illnesses from entering the picture and to achieve perfect health, the alkaline diet is the diet for you.

Thanks again for downloading this book, I hope you enjoy it!

Happy Reading.

CHAPTER 1

WHAT IS AN ALKALINE LIFESTYLE?

If you can remember back to your days in Chemistry 101, you learned the concept of alkaline and acid. There is a pH scale from 0 to 14. Pure acid is 0 and 14 is pure alkaline. So things like battery acid would be a 1 and Sodium hydroxide would be a 14. It takes 20 parts of acid to neutralize one part of alkaline.

One number that we are all aware of is our body's temperature. It is around 98.6 degrees. There is another number that most people are not aware of. That number is 7.36. That is the pH level of our blood.

Unlike our body temperature, our blood has to keep that constant rate or we would enter a condition called acidosis. Acidosis is a condition in which there is excessive acid in the body fluids. The acid would eventually burn holes in our arteries and we would die.

So why does all this matter to us?

To answer that, I have to use the following saying, "We are what we eat." If I can add to that saying, I would say, we are also what we think. I will explain that in a bit.

Let's start with what we consume. All foods have different minerals in them which make them fall somewhere in the 0 to 14 pH level. For example, take a good old can of Coke.

The pH level is about 3.4 on the scale. It is very acidic. Asparagus is about 8.5. It is Very alkaline. So when you eat these foods, the stomach starts to digest the food and the vitamins, minerals and acids start to be absorbed in the stomach, with most of the nutrients being absorbed in the small intestine. Now, our bodies need to absorb some acid.

Without it, we would not be healthy. Unfortunately, we consume a typical Western diet that is very highly acidic. We drink coffee and soda all day. We constantly test our body's ability to get rid of all this acid. Your body tries to keep up by using the alkalinity in the foods we eat. That is where the problem lies.

We eat very little alkaline foods. If your body does not get it from our foods, your body will take it from the alkaline reserves that we store in our body fluids. If that becomes depleted, your body will start to steal from your calcium based organs like your bones and brain. Sounds bad, doesn't it. You would be correct.

If all this fails, your body keeps trying to fight back. It starts to produce massive amounts of Cholesterol to surround the acid and remove it from your blood stream. And by the way, I thought I would add that it takes that acid as far away from the internal organs as possible.

Places like the Hips, butt, thighs, stomach and the back of your arms become the final resting place. Your blood vessels can only remove so much of the acid. After a while, Cholesterol starts to accumulate on the side of the walls and forms plaque.

As the acid builds up in your blood, it starts to attack the blood cells. These cells have a positive charge on the inside and a negative charge on the outside. If your cells are healthy, the negative charges are pushing other cells away. It is very much like putting 2 magnets that are negatively charged together.

They repel each other and flow freely. The acid starts to strip the negative charge away from the cell and they start to attract to each other. This is what they call blot clotting.

You start to feel lethargic and tired all the time. The clots keep much needed oxygen from flowing through the system. The clot grows and eventually finds its way to the heart or your brain. That can spell lights out.

If all of that is not bad enough, we have the concept of disease. The wonderful world of germs. We have been told that germs cause sickness. Louis Pasteur was to thank for that.

The answer is to take care of the cause and get rid of the trash. It is that simple. Disease cannot live in an healthy alkaline body. It can however live in an acidic environment. There are several ways to become more alkaline.

CHAPTER 2

WHAT IS THE ACID ALKALINE DIET?

This kind of diet has been defined in so many ways that it's hard to separate what's fact and what's made up. To put it simply, it's an eating program that involves foods that leave an alkaline residue when they're digested. It extensively promotes keeping a diet that is mostly dominated by fruits, veggies, legume, nuts, roots, and tubers.

To help us understand what makes an effective acid alkaline diet, let's take a look at the two substances that make up this diet: acid and alkaline. What is an acid?

Most of us can probably recall from high school chemistry classes that acids, by scientific definition, are substances that have several distinctive qualities: they can turn litmus paper to red, has a sour taste, and releases hydrogen ions chemically.

The strength or weakness of acidic substances are determined by the concentration of hydrogen ions. On the other hand, alkaline is the complete opposite: it turns litmus paper blue, has a bitter taste, and chemically accepts hydrogen ions. When the alkaline substance is stronger, its pH level is higher.

There are four nutrition-related acid/alkaline balance factors: the balance of acidity/alkalinity of food before they are eaten, the balance of acid and alkaline in bodily fluids and the blood, the effects of such food after they are metabolized, and the acid and alkaline chemistry of digestion.

The idea is to eat meals that include both acid and alkaline foods, as both have properties that are beneficial to the body.

The problem is, most people's eating habits are highly acid-forming. For example, sodas and coffee--which is two of the most commonly consumed drinks in the world. These two drinks are highly acidic that it can take more than 20 alkaline supplement capsules or cups of alkaline water to counteract its acidic effects.

Also, the typical diet of most people is mostly dominated by meat-and-poultry meals. Add that to the fact that consuming alkaline-forming foods is not exactly a popular choice. Acidosis happens, and catabolic damages are increased and sped up, and anabolic repairs in the body are hindered.

The best way to avoid such metabolic disasters is to keep to a sensible acid alkaline diet and eat less meat and more fruits and vegetables. Through this, the body bolsters the immune system more efficiently, plus, metabolism is improved as well. This not only gives you more energy, it helps you lose weight--and keep it off--in a healthy way.

When you stick to an eating regimen as healthy as a balanced, acid alkaline diet, you're sure to increase your energy and vitality.

CHAPTER 3

PRINCIPLES OF THE ALKALINE DIET

The alkaline diet lifestyle comprises a set of simple daily practices which easily become lifetime habits. Through the power of "the slight edge" these simple daily habits compound to produce a massive difference in terms of energy levels, wellbeing and overall health. This chapter explains the 5 key principles of the alkaline diet and how to introduce them into your life.

The alkaline diet lifestyle has gained in popularity in recent years, largely due to the influence of a number of success coaches including Anthony Robbins, who is a strong advocate and who embodies these principles.

1. Proper and effective hydration. Drinking the right amount of the right kind of water every day is the foundation of the alkaline diet lifestyle. Typically, this is 2-3 litres of alkaline, anti-oxidant rich water, which will flush out toxins and provide electro-energy to each of the trillions of cells in your body.

    Most people lose between 2 and 3 litres of fluid each day in perspiration alone and it's easy to see why the number one complaint in society is "I've got no energy". It's water your body needs - no other fluids will do. Don't overdo this however (no more than 4 litres daily), as the body needs a composition of essential salts to be healthy too.

2. In order the be fit, healthy and at an optimal weight, the blood pH (percentage hydrogen) in your body needs to be at or close to 7.365. The acid alkaline scale is logarithmic, not linear and runs from 0 (highly acidic) to 14 (highly alkaline).

    Being logarithmic means that it takes hundreds of parts of alkaline water (over pH 7) to neutralize one part of pH 2.5 cola for example). You don't need to know the science however - in just the same way as you don't need to know how electricity works in order to enjoy the benefits. Just flick the switch.

3. Ensure that your diet comprises 70% of water-rich foods which are also alkaline forming to the body. Examples include broccoli, leafy green vegetables and salads. Fruits are water-rich but many contain larger amounts of natural sugar which makes them acid forming when eaten.

    Therefore it's best to moderate the consumption of fruit. Reduce your consumption of foods and drinks which are highly acid forming, including red meat, dairy products, eggs, alcoholic and soda drinks (especially the so called "diet" varieties).

4. Thoughts can be acid or alkaline forming and will have a much greater impact on the pH of your bloodstream than anything you eat or drink. Therefore, it's very important to quiete the mind each day using meditation or some other form of relaxation.

Again, through the power of "the slight edge", the benefits of daily meditation or relaxation will compound to produce amazing results over a relatively short period of time (just a few weeks).

5. Daily alkalizing exercise is highly beneficial for the mind and the body. It's much easier than you might think too - just find a form that works for you, that you enjoy and make it a daily habit. Get into the "fat-burning" range for 20-30 minutes each day and watch the results.

Chapter 4

The Effects Of Acidity And Alkalinity On The Body

To understand the difference between acidity and alkalinity one must first understand what an alkali is. An alkali is the ionic salt of an alkaline earth metal or earth metal element. These salts have a pH of greater than 7.0 and easily dissolve in water

On the other hand, something that is acidic is derived from an acid; a chemical mixture which has a pH of less than 7.0 and, when it's dissolved in water, it produces a compound with a high hydrogen ion activity.

When we take into account the fact that everything that we eat or metabolize produces either alkaline or acidic bases into the bloodstream depending on its constituent components, as well as the fact that the human body achieves optimum performance at a pH level between 7.33 and 7.4, it makes sense to say that a diet that leans towards alkaline foods makes the most sense when we're looking to achieve optimum health.

If that is not enough, consider the fact that the human body is composed of roughly 75% water. Alkaline bases dissolve easily in, and are easily absorbed by water, unlike acidic bases which, while they break down in water, leave what is known as an "acidic residue" which can build up and eventually cause bodily functions to "slow down" (hence that tired feeling) and sometimes even to malfunction or shut down altogether.

Also, if the body's pH goes too far below 7.0 (acidic) the body will find a way to counter it. It will borrow from internal alkalinity sources, usually minerals such as calcium, magnesium or potassium which it will leech from the bones.

Depletion of calcium is one of the key causes of osteoporosis. Plaque is another problem of a diet high in acidic foods. Plaque can take the form of plaque on the teeth - but also plaque in the arteries, which is a primary contributor to heart attacks.

But even without the major concerns like osteoporosis or heart disease, high acid levels have been shown to encourage the growth of bacterial, viral or even fungal infections, all things that we could easily keep under control if we were to maintain the optimum pH balance.

Keeping all of this in mind it an alkaline diet may sound perfectly reasonable, but there is just one major problem; the average diet of western society produces high levels of acid. It is a diet that we have grown accustomed to over the last 100 years and which takes some determination to change, but once it has been adopted has proven to yield phenomenal improvements to one's overall health.

CHAPTER 5

REASONS TO GO ALKALINE AND AVOID ACIDS

The body is a marvelous tool, and its myriad processes and systems all interlock to create a streamlined machine that is designed to work without any glitches.

But as with all machines, the body needs the right kind of fuel to function properly and, when functioning properly, the waste products generated by burning this fuel are flushed out with no problem.

Perhaps once the body was perfectly balanced, and perhaps humanity once lived in a perfectly balanced world, but over the millennia we have become unbalanced; our diets and our ecosystem both becoming overwhelmed with acids and acidic wastes. The problems associated with over acidification are many and varied ranging from fatigue to arthritis to depression and even cancer.

While there is not a lot that can be done about global pollution levels, at least on an individual scale, we can control our diets and what we allow into our bodies.

Adhering to an alkaline diet may seem like it takes a lot of effort and energy, but the benefits of going and staying alkaline far outweighs the inconveniences. There are dozens of reasons to begin an alkaline diet, and it would take a book to list them all, but the top seven reasons to go alkaline and avoid acids have been listed below.

1) Weight Loss

This is a big one, for who hasn't had a weight problem at one time or another? And for those who have, what would you have given for a simple, safe and free way to lose weight?

The average western diet and lifestyle is composed of so many acid-producing substances (refined flours, sugars, meat and dairy products) and habits (smoking, alcohol consumption and prescription drug use) that our bodies have become inundated with acid wastes. And acids have a nasty way of eating into and deteriorating healthy muscle, tissues and even organs.

One of the automatic defense mechanisms of the body is to produce fat cells in order to protect our delicate organs from these excess acids. The fat cells' function is to shuttle these acid wastes away from the organs and store it in less important parts of the body, but as long as there are excess acids in the body, the fat cells will cling to the organs defensively.

Once we are able to rid ourselves of these excess acids(through maintaining a high-alkaline diet, proper hydration and exercise) the fat cells are no longer needed and the body releases them from duty, resulting in weight loss.

2) Increased Energy

The more acids that build up within the body, the less the body's natural balancing systems can process effectively, and the higher the body's acid levels become.

And the higher the acid levels become, the more alkaline minerals (calcium, magnesium, phosphates etc.) will be leached from the body's bones, muscles and tissues to make certain that the blood is able to maintain the alkaline levels necessary in order for the body to function.

When these sorts of alkaline minerals are removed efficient metabolism is inhibited, resulting in sluggishness and fatigue. The leaching of these kinds of minerals has also been linked to osteoporosis. Once the acid levels are reduced through proper diet and exercise, energy levels will increase.

3) Alleviate Allergies

An acidic environment overworks the immune system and stimulates the immune system into what is known as "response mode". The end result of this being that the body develops incredibly heightened sensitivity to all sorts of things; pollens, chemicals etc.

This heightened sensitivity we know as allergies. Some of the other ways that the body rids itself of excessive toxins and acidic wastes is through soreness, swelling, eczema and excess mucus, all things that are related to allergies. Once the excess acids have been removed from the body, the allergies and their related symptoms will disappear.

4) Reverse the Aging Process

Aging is caused by a buildup of acid wastes and the subsequent breakdown of bodily functions. When a body is too acidic a condition called acidosis occurs. Acidosis is, quite simply, the over stressing of oxidation systems and the breakdown of limpids. When this occurs it releases free radicals into the bloodstream.

Free radicals are cells that attack cell walls and membranes; killing the cell walls and membranes before finally killing the cells themselves.

When this occurs the visible result is wrinkles, poor eyesight, age spots, bad memory, fatigue, dysfunctional hormones; in short - premature aging. By removing these acids you can prevent further damage to your cells and even reverse the breakdown process.

5) Oxidation

One of the side effects of the build-up of acid wastes is that the body's cells don't get enough oxygen and this causes a slowdown in all of the cell's myriad of functions. Just like the body itself, without enough oxygen cells can die. By eliminating the acids that have been built-up in your body by changing your diet and drinking alkaline water you can re-originate your blood.

6) Decrease Blood Pressure

When a body is overly acidic the cells begin to slow down their functions (see #5) and the heart has to work all the harder to make up for their sluggishness, this causes high blood pressure.

Another side effect of high acidity is the build-up of plaque in the arteries and the decrease of the diameter of the blood vessels - which can also lead to high blood pressure. By removing the acid waste build up from your system you can improve your cell functioning and take some of the pressure off your heart.

7) Decrease Chances of Developing Degenerative Diseases

Last but not least, the build-up of acid wastes in the body (or Acidosis) is the underlying cause of almost all known degenerative diseases including (but not limited to); diabetes, obesity, liver disease, kidney disease, cardiovascular disease, neurological diseases, premature aging, hormonal imbalances, osteoporosis and even most cancers.

Degenerative diseases thrive in acidic environments, so by removing their preferred environment you can deprive them of their ability to multiply or even to take hold at all.

Chapter 6

Getting Started With The Alkaline Diet

Unless you have been oblivious of the world around, you might have heard many things about the goodness of alkaline diet and water. With so many claims, how good is this diet?

Well, unlike many of the diet charts and ideas we know of, the alkaline way of living has been influencing a lot of people, including some of the most known celebs. For starters, let's first try to understand what the concept is all about, along with the few facts that are essential for getting started.

Often called the acid ash diet, the diet mainly propagates that eating foods that are alkaline in nature will help in neutralizing the acids in the body. This simply means that pH value of the urine and blood will improve, and thereby, one can witness a lot of benefits and keep certain diseases at bay.

Under this kind of a program, you will be eating more of fresh foods and veggies, while avoiding meat, dairy and poultry. Frankly speaking, the research on the diet is limited, which is why the amount of credible evidence is also minimal. However, for people who have followed the diet, they agree to have witnessed better changes in their health.

Getting Started:

If this diet chart has inspired you, there are some elements to understand before getting started. First and foremost, you should consider the things that you can follow.

Since of the food-families are eliminated from the regular diet, you will need to understand whether your body is all the nutrients that are essential. Also, many people do have an issue leaving meat and dairy altogether, so the idea is to understand the extent to which you can follow the concept.

One of the better ideas is to replace regular water with 9.5pH alkaline water. Alkaline water is chemically processed, but it has a high pH balance and can offer the same benefits as with the diet. Keep in mind that you need to choose a brand that offers at least pH value of 9.

What are The Benefits?

Both alkaline water and diet are known to have similar kinds of benefits, but many people would rather go for high pH water instead of cutting their favorite foods.

Not to forget, drinking the water doesn't really demand and there are no side effects whatsoever- something that experts are concerned with the diet because it may miss on certain nutrients.

Some of the common benefits witnessed include natural energy boost, better hydration rate and boost in metabolism. It is also claimed that drinking water high on pH scale can help in bettering the body metabolism, which in turn can help people who are dealing with weight loss. Other claims include enhancement of all bodily functions and easy detoxification.

Our bodies need to maintain a healthy and steady alkaline to acid ratio, which is signified by the pH level of our body. The pH scale ranges from 0 to 14, and anything lower than 7 is considered acidic. Processed food items, meat and meat products, sweets, some beverages, and condiments generally produce excessive amounts of acidity in the body.

Acidosis is an abnormally high acidity level in the blood and other tissues of the body, and is the one thing that several different diseases have one thing in common. Many health experts believe that acidosis is responsible for many of the health afflictions that people suffer from today.

Alkaline, on the other hand, naturally occurs in the body to neutralize excess acidity. However, alkaline can also become depleted when our acidity levels are too high, and when we do not replenish our bodies with alkaline foods.

As mentioned earlier, acidosis leads to many health-related problems. Dangerous levels of acid get to circulate in our body and break into tissues and organs when not properly neutralized.

To prevent this, one must see to it that a healthy pH balance in the body is maintained. In order to offset the excessive amounts of acid, we need to increase our body's alkalinity.

Determining whether or not your pH levels are prevalently alkaline may be done with easy-to-use pH level strips which you can purchase in drug stores or medical supplies stores. There are pH level strips meant for testing using your saliva, and there are those for using your urine.

Basically, a saliva pH level strip will determine how much acid your body is producing; normally it is between 6.5 and 7.5 throughout the day. A urine pH level strip will tell how well you excrete excess amounts of acid; you should get between 6.0 and 6.5 in the morning and between 6.5 and 7.0 at night.

The Dangers of Excessive Acid

If you constantly experience exhaustion, headaches and having frequent colds and flu, then that could be that you have high acid levels in your body. However, the ill effects of acidosis in the body do not stop there; you might be surprised at the wide-ranging types of diseases you could get with dangerous levels of acid in your body.

Depression, hyperacidity, ulcer, skin dryness, acne and obesity are some health issues that are linked to excessive acid levels in the body. There are also those that are more serious, such as joint diseases, osteoporosis, bronchitis, frequent infections and heart diseases.

Even if you begin to take medications for these illnesses, the symptoms may be masked, but they will still continue to affect your health because you are not attacking them from their roots. Medications cause the body's acid levels to rise.

Alkaline Diet Approach

To get to the roots of these health problems, the body's pH level must be brought back to normal. There are alkaline foods that can help replenish the depleted alkaline levels in the body while neutralizing excess amounts of acid. Through an alkaline diet, sufficient amounts of alkaline are re-introduced into the body, thus bringing back the pH level to predominantly alkaline.

You can incorporate an alkaline diet into your eating habit by cutting down your intake of processed foods. These type of foods contain chemicals that only increase the acidity of your body ones they're digested.

Second, steer clear of meat and meat products, dairies and alcohol. Third, load up on fresh fruits and vegetables, as they naturally are high in alkalinity.

Even acidic fruits like oranges and lemons become alkaline after they have been digested and absorbed by the body. As a general rule, 75% of your daily food consumption should consist of alkalizing foods. The more alkaline foods we provide our bodies with, the more efficient the neutralization of excess acids will be.

CHAPTER 7

ALKALINE DIET AND ITS HEALTH BENEFITS

The food that we take today is totally different from our ancestors and is completely different from what we are so accustomed to these days. How aptly said "We are what we eat." With the advancement of technology, the types of foods we consume made us dragged along.

A view at the grocery store will shock you with aisles and aisles of processed food items and animal products. With the easy availability of fast foods nowadays, there is no difficulty in finding one in our neighborhood.

Fad diets are being partly to blame for introducing a whole new eating habits, this include high-protein diets. In recent years, consumption of animal products and refined food items have increased as more and more people leave out the daily supply of fruits and vegetables in their diets.

It comes as no surprise why, these days, many people are suffering from different types of ailments and allergies such as bone diseases, heart problems and many others. Some health experts link these diseases to the type of foods we eat.

There are certain types of food that disrupts the balance in our body that, during such instances, health problems arise. If only we could modify our eating habits, it's unlikely that prevention of diseases and restoration of health can be achieved.

For a healthy body, the alkaline and acid ration must be balanced, which is measured by the pH level in the body. pH values range from 0 to 14 and 7 is considered neutral.

Any value less than 7 is considered acidic. Refined food, such as meat and meat derivatives, candies and some sweetened drinks usually generate great amount of acid for the body.

Acidosis, a case of high level of acidic in the blood stream and body cells is the common index for the current different diseases inflicting many people. Some health professionals conclude that acidosis is responsible for the critical diseases suffered by many individuals nowadays.

Alkaline or alkaline diet, which normally present in our body neutralize the high level of acidic in the body to achieve equilibrium state. This is the main function of the alkaline in the body. However, the presence of the alkaline in the body is quickly depleted due to the high level of acidic contents it has to neutralize and there is insufficient alkaline food consumed to replenish the loss alkaline.

As described previously, acidosis causes many health-related problems. Critical level of acid get into our system, breaking the cells and organs when not neutralize properly. To prevent this, one must see to it that a balance pH is maintained.

To test whether our body contains higher level of alkaline can be carried out with ease. This with the use of a pH strips which are obtainable from any pharmacy. There are two types of strips, one for the saliva and the other for urine.

Generally, a saliva pH level strip will determine the level of acid your body is producing; the normal values should be between 6.5 and 7.5 throughout the day. A urine pH level strip will show the level of acid; a normal reading should be between 6.0 and 6.5 in the morning and between 6.5 and 7.0 at night

High Level of Acidity Is Harmful for the Body

If you consistently suffer from fatigue, headaches and having regular common cold and flu, these symptoms indicate a high level of acid in the body. The effect of acidosis in the body not only inhibits the normal diseases that we know but other diseases that you may suffer is caused by high level of acid in the body.

Depression, high acidity, ulcer, dry skin, acne and overweight are some of those linked with extreme level of acidity in our body. Not limiting to these, other critical and serious diseases such as joint diseases, osteoporosis, bronchitis, frequent infections and heart diseases.

Even with medications, the symptoms may be disguised and continue to affect your health as the root of the problem has not been completely eradicated. Taking more medicine will only compound the problem as the anti-inflammatory medicine will add to the acidic level in the body.

In order to reach the root of the diseases, our systems pH value must be maintained in a healthy state. Naturally occurring alkaline foods are able to supplement the lost alkaline levels in the body during the neutralizing process.

By maintaining a healthy alkaline diet, sufficient amount of alkaline are replenished in the system thereby bringing the body back to the predominant alkaline state.

So what are the ways to include an alkaline diet into our eating habits? The very basic first step is to reduce the amount of refined food intake. As we already know, these foods contain many chemicals which are the culprits in increasing the acidic level in our body.

The next step is to cut down on the intake of meat and their derivatives and also the amount of liquor. The final step is to increase the amount of fresh fruits and vegetables, as they are naturally high in alkalinity

The higher the amount of alkaline foods we put into our system, the greater the neutralization of the acidic condition in our body.

CHAPTER 8

Guidelines To Maintaining A Healthy Alkaline Balance

Many people are not aware of how important the foods that they eat are to their health and wellbeing. Foods can be either alkaline or acidic in nature. What determines if a food is alkaline or acidic? This is determined in part, by the amount of "ash residue" that exists once you have consumed a particular food and it has been fully digested.

The higher the ash content the more acidic the food is. The higher the mineral content, the more alkaline the food would be. Therefore, if a food has a higher ash content it is more acidic and consuming a lot of acidic foods will eventually weaken your health and immune system.

The ideal diet to follow is one that is 80% alkaline and 20% acidic. However, in the United States, the very opposite is true. We consume a diet that averages out to be 80% acidic and only 20% alkaline.

If we try to follow a more alkaline diet we will not only achieve better health but we can help to correct nutritional deficiencies and get many poor health issues under control.

It is also important to note that in addition to your body becoming more alkaline through the proper food choices, you can also achieve more alkalinity by your lifestyle choices.

For example, stress can make your body much more acidic. If you are continually experiencing stress you will tend to be more acidic even if you eat more alkaline foods.

The body is a wonderfully complex mechanism that responds to everything that we do to it in either in a positive or negative way. The brain-body connection should not therefore be overlooked when you are trying to create a more alkaline balance in your body.

The Acid Alkaline Equation:

For the human body to function at its best, the ideal alkalinity should be between 7.0 to 8.0 pH. pH is an abbreviation for "power of hydrogen". Anything below a 7.0ph would be considered acidic. Obviously the lower that number, the more acidic your body would be.

The normal pH level of human blood should be at around 7.4. If the blood pH falls below 6.8 or goes above 7.8 it can be very dangerous because the body's cells will not be able to function properly and can be potentially life threatening.

The natural process of the metabolism is to produce a certain amount of acid. This is why it is very important to eat as much alkaline foods as you can in order for your body to not develop an acidic state.

How Alkaline Foods Can Help Reverse the Disease Process:

Many diseases can develop when a body is in an acidic state. For example, cancer cells will thrive in an acidic environment and disease can proliferate in such a state. Another common problem that can develop is osteoporosis because when a body is acidic it is lacking sufficient calcium which is an alkalizing mineral.

So clearly being in an acidic state can contribute to poor health and the onset of various disease conditions. A body that is alkaline has the ability to regenerate more quickly and remove excess toxins more efficiently than an acidic body.

Human beings were truly meant to consume a more alkaline diet and prior to only the past few recent decades has man eaten such an acidic diet. Traditionally we have eaten predominantly whole fresh foods including an abundance of fruits and vegetables.

An unfortunate trend in our modern society has been to consume large amounts of processed foods which have contributed to the increase in diseases that proliferate today.

Some Food Guidelines for Alkalinity:

There are many wonderful foods that you can choose from that are alkaline and can help your health and vitality. Raw foods of course, such as fresh fruits and vegetables are among the most alkaline foods you can consume.

In this whole state, you are supplying your body with vital nutrition and enzymes that will nourish your cells and help strengthen your immune system, protecting you from degenerative disease development.

Some other top alkalinizing foods include; fresh fruits and vegetables, raw nuts and seeds, sprouted grains and plenty of fresh clean water. Try to limit your intake of processed foods, artificial sweeteners, dairy products and eat meat proteins in moderation.

A simple and very effective way to increase your alkalinity is to add a green drink to your daily diet. There are many high quality products on the market to choose from.

Reduce your intake of acidic foods.

Examples of these types of foods include all processed foods, fast foods, any white flour products and dairy products. Also incorporate neutral balanced foods which are neither acidic nor alkaline such as brown rice and whole wheat products in moderation.

And of course, drink plenty of water. By following these guidelines you should be able to create and maintain a healthy alkaline balance in your body and help to prevent the onset of disease by maintaining a strong and balanced immune system.

CHAPTER 9

HOW TO IMPROVE THE ALKALINITY OF YOUR BODY AND BE HEALTHIER

You have to improve the alkalinity of your body to combat the symptoms of premature aging. Be sure to follow a strict diet and an exercise habit to help you gain back the explosive energy of youth.

If you are 25 to 30 years old and you always feel low on energy, you better be careful because you may be acidic. An acidic body can lead to headaches, anemia, aches and pains in your muscles and joints. High acidic levels in the body can also cause major illnesses like cancer and acute diabetes.

When I speak of acidity, we refer to that state of your inner terrain where it is under imbalance. Just imagine a rain forest where there are more predators than prey. The jungle will not survive because the ecosystem is at an imbalance. Same for our bodies, we will feel sick and fatigued if our inner ecosystem is at an imbalanced state.

Unfortunately, western diet has been known to be very acidic. This means that in order to feel healthier than you are now, you have to invest some time and will power to changing your lifestyle and your food intake.

Change of lifestyle includes incorporating exercise in your daily routine. Exercise is very effective to help you gain back the energy that you lost.

Exercise also makes you strong and fit to perform your job and other daily tasks.

Find a fun exercise and with a positive attitude, you have to stick with it. You will always need to have a positive attitude so you can accomplish a lot of hard tasks that you think you can't.

Always say that you can and do some activities that will help reinforce a can do attitude. Engaging in sports, for example, can help you develop a can do attitude.

You must also change the alkalinity of your body. This can be achieved if you eat a balanced alkaline diet. You do not have to change your lifestyle, and you do not need to go completely vegetarian. Just follow the alkaline food chart so you can keep track of all your food intake.

If you keep track of your food intake, you will surely have a balanced alkalinity of body that will make you healthier. With a balanced inner terrain, you will not feel the aches and pains or the low energy and fatigue.

You will have a balanced alkalinity in your body to make feel younger and stronger. It is guaranteed to make you perform at the peak of your energy.

USING A LIST OF PH OF FOODS FOR HEALTH, ENERGY AND WEIGHT

To maintain a healthy body and mind, the pH of foods that you eat daily must be balanced. To call your meal balanced it should consist of alkaline and acid in a proportionate ratio. A healthy body houses 80% alkalinity and 20% acidity. Too much acid in food items can cause stomach discomfort and temporary instability in the body.

The Alkaline content in our food keeps the body mechanism in order. It not only prevents diseases but also cures them naturally. If you can, go on a perfectly pH balanced diet for a while and see how much your health improves. Alkaline cleanses the body flushing the toxins and harmful chemicals from the body.

It strengthens the immune system in your body and keeps viruses and bacteria at bay. You call a food item healthy when the acid and the alkaline level in it are balanced. Too much acid or fats can play host to a number of health problems such as weight gain, acidity, fatigue, heartburn and mental stress.

Which food items are alkaline?

Eat plenty of green vegetables and fruits. Depending on the seasonal availability of the greens include them raw or cooked in your daily diet. See that the pH in the foods you eat is 80% alkaline. You can also have many other vegetables like turnips, eggplants, tomatoes, turnips to increase the alkaline level in the body.

However, take care some of these vegetables turn acid by eating some of them cooked. Spinach is an alkaline veggie when eaten raw, but when cooked becomes acidic. The tip of asparagus is acidic, so cut it off before using.

Fresh salads, fruits, juices and vegetable broths are the best alkaline foods. Besides fresh vegetables and fruits, eat lots of almonds, wheatgrass and sprouts. Include fresh fruits such as bananas, lemons, oranges, melons, apples and dates in your breakfast.

Acid Vs Alkaline

Acid and Alkaline act in opposite ways. While the alkaline content serves as a shield to protect the body from diseases, too much acid content creates diseases. Too much acidic food makes your skin look old and wrinkled. Oily, fried and fatty foods are full of acid, which creates heartburn due to their acidity. Acids slow down the process of vitamin and nutrient absorption by the body.

The acid forms a coating on the walls of the intestines disabling the functions of the part. Due to this, toxins build up and start hindering the functions of the body. Alkaline foods add benefit to your health in many ways.

They enhance the absorption of cells and allow smooth movement of the energy particles. They improve the antioxidant production, which improves the looks of the skin, prevents colds, headaches and seasonal infections.

They reduce the overgrowth of yeast and parasites within the body. Due to regulated digestion and other functions in the body, alkalinity in the body allows you peaceful sleep and complete relaxation.

Adding to all benefits, the pH of foods increases the lifespan of a person and keeps you fit. Those who wish to lose pounds can stay on a healthy pH diet and look slim and attractive.

You can feel the difference when you balance the pH in your diet and lead a healthy lifestyle. If you can't do 80%, keep the alkaline level of your body at around least 60% and acidity at 40%. Avoid fatty foods and red meat if you want to stabilize your alkaline levels.

CHAPTER 11

ACID-ALKALINE FOODS

There are many foods that have been available in the market. And these foods are not all good for us. Choosing the right foods for us is very essential. Acid alkaline foods should be our basis in choosing them.

Alkaline diet has been popular for the wonders it brings to the body. It is a kind of diet wherein the basis is the maintenance of balanced pH condition inside your body. Alkaline foods are the ones that are good for your body. On the other hand, acid foods are bad for your health.

How do we know what are the acid and alkaline foods?

Acid foods consist of red meats, pasta, rice, sweets, frizzy, alcohols, caffeine and others. Pork, beef, chicken, turkey and lamb are the examples of red meats that are harmful for our health.

Alcohols are very bad for our livers. They cause liver cancer. Cigarettes do not do good for our health too. They cause lung cancer.

Many people, even at their early ages, really want to drink alcohols and enjoy smoking. They keep on doing these things because they are not yet experiencing the bad effects that can be gotten from these stuffs.

However, time will come that your health will suffer because of the accumulation of nicotine from cigars and chemicals from alcohols that are detrimental to our health.

We must know how to prevent ourselves from these unwanted habits. It really is true that avoiding yourself from these kinds of stuff is hard. So, the best thing we can do is to substitute them with drinking root beer or eating chewing gums.

You just need time to practice preventing these things until they are totally gone out of your system. Not only this, you should avoid eating processed foods and using artificial sweeteners.

As times pass by, people are getting used to accumulating so much unwanted chemicals from processed foods. We are deceived that we will lose weight when we use artificial sweeteners. This is not true.

Losing weight is easily obtained by eating alkaline foods. Alkaline foods are really beneficial in losing weight, having a healthy lifestyle and maintaining a good, young looking personality.

Not only this, but you can also have a more stable emotional condition and better mind capability. We tend to be emotional when we don't feel good. It is when we feel aches and pains.

People are aware that fruits and vegetables are good. These are alkaline foods. Alkaline foods include fruits such as avocado, lime, lemon, apple, banana, watermelon and papaya. Vegetables such as squash, broccoli, cauliflower and potatoes with peels are alkaline forming foods too.

To maintain our natural ph balance of 7.4 we need to eat 80% alkaline foods. But to eat alkaline foods we must know what the various alkaline forming foods are. By consuming these alkalizing foods we will be able to carve our road to good health and a long life.

Alkaline forming foods are mostly vegetables and fruits. Green vegetables are higher on the chart of alkaline foods. Broccoli, asparagus, cabbage, lettuce, miso, leeks are all alkaline vegetables. Even vegetables like carrots, tomatoes and potatoes with their peel all help with alkalizing.

Spinach is a tricky one, if uncooked it is fine and helps with alkalinity but if we cook spinach it helps make acid. So one should try and consume spinach raw. Asparagus tips that are white are acidic and should be snipped away.

Fruits like melons, mangoes, apples and bananas all help form alkaline ash. Even lemons which are acidic in their nature are actually alkalizing foods since the effect that they have on the body is alkaline.

Fruits and vegetables are all alkaline forming food but care should be taken that they are cleaned thoroughly before consumption so as not to consume harmful chemicals along with these benefits.

Even though vegetables and fruits are alkaline forming foods they are not the only ones. Olive oil is a high alkaline forming food and one should try and cook all their food in it. Other oils such as vegetable oils and fats like butter are bad and acidic foods.

Avocado butter is an alkaline forming food and should be substituted for normal butter. In fact milk and milk products are acidic and should be avoided.

Almonds are alkaline forming food and are also power houses of energy. People of all ages should have a few almonds everyday.

Honey also helps restore the alkaline/acid balance and has great healing powers. For a sour throat try some honey with lemon and ginger and you will feel the difference instantly. Garlic is excellent at helping with alkalinity. Try and add garlic to most of your recipes.

For those who like their beverages a word of advice stay away from coffee and tea. These are acidic foods. Alkaline forming beverages are herbal teas, coffee substitutes and fresh lemon water. These can be safely consumed without harming the body or exposing it to diseases.

On the other hand, sodas and alcoholic drinks are highly acidic foods. One should consume fresh foods as opposed to processed foods since the latter is acidic in nature. Processed foods are all bad for the body and should be avoided completely.

But another very important requirement of the body is water. Normal water does not benefit the body as much as alkalizing water does. Alkalizing water, as the name suggests, helps form alkaline and so is greatly beneficial to the body.

Consuming about 6 to 8 glasses of alkaline water is very healthy for the body and also helps maintain the ph balance so keeping the body away from all the diseases as well preventing cell degeneration. Alkaline forming foods are the best gifts we can give our bodies. Only they can help the body develop a strong immune system.

CHAPTER 12

TOP 10 MOST ALKALINE FOODS FOR YOUR DIET

Everything, living or non-living, is either acidic or alkaline. However, humans are creatures made to consume alkaline foods and stand as an alkaline organism in the food chain.

Our blood's pH level is pretty much determined by the food we eat. And with our blood being non-alkaline, or simply, acidic, our body will poorly perform and will have difficulty in resisting the harsh effects of oxidation and disease-inflicting viruses.

Here are the Top 10 Alkaline Foods that will give your mind and body more health and energy:

1. **Avocados, Bananas (ripe), Berries, Carrots, Celery, Currants, Dates, Garlic.**

These foods are very high in antioxidants. They have a pH value of 8.0. They chemically react to acidic foods of pH 5.0 and elevate them near the alkaline levels. Berries, dates and especially garlic have special properties that regulate blood pressure as well.

2. Apples (sweet), Apricots, Alfalfa sprouts.

These ones are super digestible foods, which are high in fiber and have a pH value of 8.0. They are also rich in enzymes that are helpful in maintaining the body's hormonal balance.

Surely, an apple a day keeps the doctor away. Don't forget to include apricots though. For those who do not know, Alfalfa sprouts are those sprouting seeds of beans that are commonly mixed in salads and sandwiches.

3. Grapes (sweet), Passion fruit, Pears (sweet), Pineapple, Raisins, Umeboshi plum, Vegetable juices.

At a pH of 8.5, this group is high in antioxidants and vitamins A, B and C. Grapes, raisins and plums are blood-regulating foods, which lower blood pressure and the risks of getting a heart disease.

Pineapple, on one hand, is rich in L-Carnitine, which uses body fat as an energy source and is good for trimming that growing waistline. Vegetable juices, on the other hand, are high in iron and good for cellular detoxification.

4. Chicory, Kiwifruit, Fruit juices.

They have natural sugar that doesn't form acidic compounds during digestion. Rather, these foods have alkaline-forming properties that give more energy to the body.

Still at a pH level of 8.5, this group is rich in flavonoids, a chemical compound in natural foods that have antioxidant properties. Kiwi fruit even has higher Vitamin C content than oranges. Chicory, a bitter-tasting close relative of the lettuce, also has insulin that supports the pancreas and aids the body in preventing diabetes.

5. Watercress, Seaweeds, Asparagus.

With a pH level of 8.5, this group is unique as a powerful acid reducer. Watercress, for example, is called the natural super food. It is the first leafy vegetable consumed by human beings and is commonly prepared as part of a healthy salad.

It is best eaten raw and it contains lots of iron and calcium like seaweeds. Asparagus is even more special for its highest content of asparagines, an amino acid important to the nervous system.

6. Limes, Mango, Melons, Papaya, Parsley.

This food group has a pH of 8.5 and is best at cleansing the kidneys. Papaya is even the healthiest laxative that promotes defecation and colon cleansing. Parsley, the most popular herb, is the best dirt sweeper of the intestines when taken raw. It is also a diuretic, which is necessary in cleaning the kidneys. Limes, mangoes and melons are vitamin-rich fruits that are alkaline-forming during digestion.

7. Cantaloupe, Cayenne (Capsicum).

The group with the most alkaline reactive properties among the foods with the pH of 8.5, they are high in enzymes needed by the endocrine system. Cayenne has antibacterial properties and is also high in Vitamin A, which is essential in fighting free radicals that causes stress and illnesses. Cantaloupes, a relative of melons, is very low in sugar but high in fiber.

8. Agar Agar (Organic Gelatin)

Still with a pH of 8.5, Agar Agar is a gelatin substitute made from seaweeds that is high in iron and calcium as well. It is very digestible and has the highest fiber content among all foods.

9. Watermelon.

At a pH level of 9.0, Watermelon are very alkaline. Because of its high fiber and water content at 92% of its entire weight, watermelon is a mild diuretic and a great source of beta-carotene, lycopene and vitamin C. This thirst-quenching fruit is the most life and energy supporting food when used in a week-long fasting and colon cleansing.

10. Lemons.

At the top of the list is the Amazing Lemon. With its electrolytic properties and a pH level of 9.0, lemons are considered the most alkalizing food. It is the most potent and most immediate relief for colds, cough, flu, heartburns, hyperacidity and other virus-related ailments. Lemons are natural antiseptic that disinfects and heals wounds. It is also the best liver tonic that detoxifies and energizes the liver.

CHAPTER 13

ALKALIZING OUR BODIES WITH FRESH FRUITS AND VEGETABLES

Many experts are now even recommending between 5 and 13 servings of fruits and veggies every day to help prevent disease and illness. Frequent consumption of produce can help keep High Blood pressure, Cancer, Heart Disease, Cataracts, and many other illnesses at bay. Why are we, as a nation, so reluctant to incorporate these disease-preventing and vitality-creating substances into our lives?

Years ago our Parents and Grandparents enjoyed diets full of quality fruits and vegetables, on an everyday basis. It certainly wouldn't have surprised anyone to even see two separate vegetables cooked with every dinner.

Today, it's a feat in itself to even find a home cooked meal. In many Third World countries, they still continue to consume fresh produce more often than they do dairy or meat products, and many of the same countries have a much lower rate of Cancers, Diabetes, and Autoimmune diseases. T

hese facts should certainly make an inquisitive person wonder, "Why is the richest, most advanced country in the World, the United States of America, also one of the sickest countries in the World?"

One answer to that question is that our hectic and very industrialized way of living has made fresh produce and whole foods a thing of the past for many Americans.

If we do take the time to add fruits and veggies to our daily intake, it is often in the form of canned foods, sugary juices, or preserved frozen varieties; which are quick and easy, but retain very little nutritional value.

Most of us do know that we have to make a conscious effort to include more produce in our diets, but how many people actually understand that the quality of the fruit and vegetable is equally as important as the consumption?

One reason that fruits and vegetables are such powerful healers is that they help to Alkaline the body; or restore the body's blood PH level to a non-acidic level. One of the primary reasons why our bodies become infested with pain, illness, and disease, is because our PH (Potential Hydrogen) systems are severely out of balance. Now, what is this PH system all about?

The PH balance of the blood stream is one of the most important biochemical balances in all of human body chemistry. Everything single system in your body is affected by your PH level...

Your PH is measured on a scale from 0 to 14. The higher the number on the scale, the more alkaline the substance, and the lower the number the more acidic the substance.

Healthy human blood normally remains around a slightly alkaline 7.3. When levels drop below this number, blood becomes more acidic and an environment of disease and illness can develop.

The effect that foods and drinks have on our bodies is measured after digestion. They become either acid-forming or alkaline-forming.

Many of the foods and drinks that are part of our North American diet are acid forming, and can lead to Acidosis, which is a condition that often leads to permanent cell damage. Some examples of acid-forming and alkaline-forming foods are as follows:

Alkaline forming: most fruits, green vegetables, peas, beans, lentils, spices, herbs and seasonings, and seeds and nuts. It's certainly no coincidence that most Alkaline foods are fruits and vegetables. These foods were created to be the foundation of our diets, not the side dishes.

Acid forming: meat, fish, poultry, eggs, grains, and legumes. These choices dominate our American diets.

How raw fruits and vegetables heal and prevent illness with enzymes

While eating cooked fruits and vegetables may still provide some Alkalizing benefit, the majority of the healing power of produce exists within the enzymes that are present in raw fruits and veggies. The role of enzymes is to speed up the rate of every chemical reaction in every single cell of your body.

In order for minerals, vitamins, hormones, and herbs to do their jobs, they need the assistance of enzymes to reach the intended cells in an effective manner. In fact, Enzymes are often called the "source of life".

By ingesting raw fruits and vegetables, enzymes are present in amounts sufficient to aid in the digestion process, without depleting the body's enzyme stores. As digestion is effectively completed, and waste eliminated, acidity is also reduced and the body moves towards Alkalinity.

Eating fruits and vegetables that are high in enzymes can help to increase your energy levels, as well as potentially aid weight loss, rejuvenate skin, and generally support overall health. Fruits and vegetables high in enzymes not only keep our bodies healthy and restore vitality, but they also can be very pleasing to our palates as well.

The most important point of this chapter to remember is to increase your servings of fruits and vegetables every day, and more often than not consume them in the raw state. Compliance with this simple rule will help keep you disease, illness, and pain-free for a very long time.

CHAPTER 14

EXAMINING GOOD FOOD WITH ALKALINE DIET CHART

If you're not familiar with what it is, the chart presents different food and beverages, the category in which a food/beverage belongs, and the level of alkaline or acid it contains. Why should you examine the alkalinity and acidity of the food you eat?

Our body contains both acid and alkaline chemicals. Keeping our body's pH or acid-alkaline levels in a balance is the key to staying strong and healthy.

Once our body is overpowered by excessive acidity, we will feel weaker and less active. In time, the continuous increase of acidity in our system will give way to premature signs of aging and the development of chronic illnesses. Below are the common effects of over-acidity:

- Muscle and joint pains

- Headaches

- Nausea

- Fatigue

- Unexplained Weakness

- Difficulty in Breathing

- Dizziness

- Heart palpitations

- Cramps

If you notice that you are often experiencing any of the above symptoms, it may have something to do with your diet. Perhaps it's time to take an objective look about your way of eating and see if you can change it for the better.

If you have been eating a lot of highly acidic foods, this is the perfect opportunity for you to start making better food choices to improve your health condition.

Why Use An Alkaline Diet Chart

There are foods that contain low to very high levels of acid. Examples of highly acidic food and beverage are pork, beef, veal, shellfish, coffee, tea, soda, beer and liquor. Artificial sweeteners may seem like "good sweets" but these synthetic products actually contain very high acid.

People, especially those who are on a diet should be particularly careful about their choice of snacks. Just because a certain snack says low fat and no sugar doesn't mean it's good for you. Remember, these snacks contain artificial sweeteners which have high acid content.

Then, there are foods that are considered to be very good for us because of their alkaline content. Fresh vegetables like broccoli, raw spinach, lettuce, celery, and parsley; fruits like papaya, kiwi, apples and pears; and natural sweeteners like honey, maple syrup and rice syrup are known to be wonderful alkaline sources.

Using an alkaline diet chart will make it easier for you to decide which foods you want to include in your diet.

51

CHAPTER 15

TOP WAYS TO ACHIEVE ALKALINE PH IN YOUR BODY

An alkaline pH is live oxygen for the body. If we do not get enough oxygen within minutes we will die. Similarly if we are derived of an alkaline pH in time we will die. So if we want to lead healthy and long lives then the answer lies in achieving and maintaining an alkaline pH of the body.

The neutral pH rests at 7 and more than this is alkaline while lesser is an acidic pH. The human body naturally has a pH of 7.4. This is alkaline. Our high pH is of utmost importance for the acidic functions of the body to continue smoothly.

Since all the metabolic activities of the body releases toxins and waste they are acidic in nature, if the pH of the body is also acidic they will not be balanced out and so diseases will occur.

An alkaline pH on the other hand helps to flush the toxins out of the body as well as carry oxygen to the parts of the body. Most diseases have their roots in an acid environment.

When our pH tilts to the acidic side the consequences are serious diseases like arthritis, coronary problems, migraines, cancer and so on. Even seemingly small problems like constipation and common colds have an acid pH to blame for.

The next question is how to maintain this alkaline pH. Whatever comes in contact with our body has an effect on us. Even chemicals and air which come in contact with our skin and hair affect us. We must try to introduce our body to only those things which have a positive effect on the body. We are most affected by what we eat and drink.

By consuming alkalizing foods we will be able to maintain as well as restore our alkaline pH while on the other hand acidic foods will unbalance this body pH and lead to serious complications.

Alkaline foods consist of mainly vegetables and fruits. Green vegetables like broccoli, cabbage, salad leaves and asparagus are very high alkalizing foods.

Not only do they help to maintain an alkaline pH but also provide roughage for the body and so help in releasing toxins and wastes of the body. Vegetables and fruits are best eaten raw. Cooking leads to vegetables losing their nutrients. Spinach when eaten raw is highly alkalizing for the body but the same leaves when cooked become acidic in nature.

Care should be taken in washing the fruits and vegetables well so as to not consume harmful pesticides etc with them. Other foods like almonds, honey, olive oil, miso, herbal teas and alkaline water should also form a major part of our diet if an alkaline pH is to be maintained.

Acidic foods like wheat, barley, animal flesh, processed foods and juices should be taken off the menu. It takes 32 glasses of ordinary water to balance out the acid introduced in out body by on glass of soda.

An alkaline pH will safeguard us from all kinds if disease, will prevent cell degeneration as well as energize us.

CHAPTER 16

TIPS TO MAKE THE ALKALINE DIET SUCCESSFUL FOR YOU

Success refers to that feeling of accomplishment after one struggle in your life. In any way we can, we always strive to be successful in everything we do. We just have to push the limits or go beyond what we think we can do. Going on an alkaline diet can be your health struggle to lead you to weight loss success.

You might think that learning the hardest way is always the best way to get rid of acidic foods that make you unhealthy. Don't take this too seriously, though. It will be easiest if you pay attention to these tips on how the starvation plan will ensure a thriving lifestyle for the rest of your days.

This cut-down involves 80% of your total regular food intake. Eating a lot of fruits and vegetables is the easiest way to meet this cut-down, but don't limit yourself to these two food groups. There are other ways to successfully accomplish your plan.

- Drink a lot of water and citrus-rich juices. Squeeze a tangerine or a lemon into a glass of water habitually. Lemonades are must-haves when undergoing successfully the reducing

- Instead of bread, treat yourself to sautéed or salad vegetables. Prepare a huge bowl of large cabbage or broccoli salad since these vegetables help intensify your body's pH level.

- Have fresh apples or peaches. As much as possible, do away with snacks that have higher amount of acid substances.

- Eat fish and lamb as substitutes for the usual pork or beef

- Chicken, cooked in various ways, can also serve as a healthy alternative for meaty viands.

- Deputize Millet or Quinoa for wheat-enriched foods. Avoid eating white bread since they have high levels of acid.

- Add greenish food supplements such as Miso and Broth to any dish. Both of these ingredients help invigorate the alkaline levels of your body.

CHAPTER 17

GETTING ALKALINE WITH COOL SHORTCUTS

The concept of "Getting Alkaline" is not the latest health fad, or some trend that will disappear any time soon. It is gaining traction consistently and methodically in the marketplace, and the concept is so fundamental and common sense to health conscious people that they usually have an aha. experience as soon as they hear about it.

As we grow and are exposed to acidic foods, stress, pollution, chemicals and even natural acids like lactic acid, our bodies become acidic. Everything we eat and drink has either an acid or alkalizing effect.

Think of it like a bank account and everything you take into your body is either an alkaline deposit or an acidic withdrawal. For example, soda is a huge withdrawal; green and yellow vegetables and alkaline water are excellent deposits.

When our body is acidic bad things happen. Diseases flourish in acidic environments. Some doctors and nutritionists believe that maintaining a healthy PH balance makes you immune to diseases, even cancer.

Eating an alkaline diet offers benefits like:

Your body will adjust to its natural weight -You will have increased energy

Better sleep patterns

You will gain lean muscle

Drastically lower risk of illness (some claim you can't get sick at all.)

So how do you do it? Here are 7 cool shortcuts to help you get there:

1. Get a PH test kit and measure your PH level regularly. Just by measuring regularly you start to see patterns, and know what things affect your body either positively or negatively. These test kits are inexpensive, and are readily available at your local health food store.

2. Add alkaline water to your diet. This has had more impact for me personally than any other single thing. Hydration itself is critical to getting alkaline, and most people don't drink enough water. Those that do drink lots of water would get a huge boost in alkalinity they drank alkaline water.

    To determine how much water you should be drinking, just divide your body weight in two and drink that many ounces of alkaline water a day. In other words, a 180 pound man should drink at least 90 ounces of water a day. Then add an alkalizing supplement, and watch how quickly you see positive health improvements.

3. Start each day with a glass of fresh lemon juice. Just take a lemon or two and squeeze the juice into a glass of water. Although lemons are acidic, they have a strong alkalizing effect on your body, as well as good digestive benefits. A little tart at first, but once you're used to it you will learn to love it.

4. Just add salad. Add a salad to your lunch and dinner every day. Spinach salad is particularly good, but almost all green and yellow vegetables are alkalizing. Also, adjust the portion size on your plate. Cut down on the meat, potatoes and gravy, and increase the serving size of your veggies. Not hard to do, but it makes a big difference.

5. Cut back on refined sugar. We already know sugar isn't good for us, but it also causes acidity in our bodies. Understanding that, become a label reader, and check how many grams of sugar are in what you're about to eat.

6. **Add "Super Alkalizers" to your alkaline diet:**

    Greens like Kale, Mustard Greens, and Broccoli

    Millet or Quinoa instead of wheat

    Fish and lamb over beef

    Olive oil instead of other vegetable oils

    Miso broth. Just dissolve one teaspoon of miso into a cup of hot, not boiling water.

    Use fresh garlic in your cooking

7. Add supplements. Enzymes, ionic form minerals, and vitamins A and D are particularly good at helping the body maintain a healthy pH level.

CHAPTER 18

ALKALINITY AS THE SWEET LIFE

Because we now realize that our bodies function ideally when they are just slightly alkaline it becomes helpful to balance our bodily pH level within that range.

The bottom line is that all research reveals that disease flourishes in an acid environment,including cancers. Most health authorities state that a long-term overly acidic body condition effectively diminishes the effectiveness of our immune system and generally results in chronic inflammation and disease.

It is obvious that you must find your current pH level to begin to help yourself. This is the baseline that you must try to change for the better. An excellent and inexpensive way to quickly show your pH level is to buy ordinary litmus paper, found in most health stores.

A paper scale typically come with the product that defines, by color codes, the real pH of the saliva or urine. Insert a small strip of the paper under your tongue and or in your urine, preferably upon waking.

Normally saliva pH levels are at 7 or 7.5. Higher that these is increasingly alkaline, lower is acid.

Once you've established that you need to make a change in your pH level you can search out alkaline or acid specific foods to help correct your levels.

These can readily be found on the web (Google + alkaline foods or acid foods) There are even handy charts for you to print out for your shopping trips.

The body's composition consists of 70 % water. The most vital fluid within your body is blood. Then logically we can conclude that blood is mainly water. All of your musculature, skin and vital organs need massive amounts of water in order for them to work optimally.

Water is the vehicle by which oxygen is transported to your cells. It removes waste and delivers energy. Drinking adequate supplies of pH tested water is vital to optimal health levels. Adding lemon juice or some other alkaline fruit to flavor water boost overall alkalinity.

With a little bit of your own research you'll discover supplements that you can use daily to boost alkaline levels or acid levels as your specific needs dictate. To consistently keep up your alkalinity you will find specific things that you'll be wise to stop using and also things that you must begin to use regularly.

What to Avoid.

Artificial sweeteners typically are very acidic and have adverse effects on your nervous and digestive systems. (Sucralose, Nutrisweet, saccharin). A number of these sweeteners have additionally been linked cancer.

Stay away from red meats, most of these red meat are extremely acidic and also have real low water content. Better to substitute chicken, turkey, fish to give us the protein we need.

Reduce your supply of processed and refined foods such as flour, preservatives and food coloring. These foods are known to leave acid residues in the body. Further, these chemicals are stored in the fat cells.

Stay away from fatty and fried foods, they also raise acid levels.

Alcohol increases the acid levels in our body and should be avoided. Additionally it significantly increases acid levels in blood. Make increased alkaline water levels the health alternative to alcohol, remember to add lemon.

Stress is a major culprit. It raises acid levels and blood pressure while also increasing adrenaline into the blood stream. It also causes the stomach to generate greater levels of acids. you should counter the effects of stress with exercise, it boosts alkalinity.

Achieving optimizing levels of alkalinity is imperative to good health. Diagnosis and treatment of pH are relatively easy and inexpensive and available to all. Your sweetness factor is up to you.

Conclusion

Over the last 50 to 60 years, our diet has changed. We no longer eat a natural diet from the garden or the local farm. Canned, frozen, packaged, processed, and fast foods are now readily available and have been increasing in our diet since the 1950's.

Because of our busy and fast pace life, many people are eating these "convenience" foods in their daily diet. During this time, diseases are also increasing, and new diseases are manifesting every year.

Many people think that diet is something they do to lose weight or to keep a disease in control such as heart disease, or diabetes. Diet is simply eating and drinking the right foods that provide optimum nutrition to fuel the body so it can thrive and be healthy.

What you put in your mouth is a choice you make and when your choices are causing you to suffer, as in poor health, you can change these choices and it will change the outcome you experience.

Food is necessary to feed the cells in your body and keep them healthy. However, many people have abused the true meaning of why they eat food. They eat for social and emotional reasons, because of food addictions and cravings.

They eat too much of the wrong kind of foods that cause excess weight and poor health. The right kind of protein, carbohydrate, and fat together with the right balance with each meal will bring about better health and weight loss.

What you eat is only part of maintaining good health. Negative thoughts, physical and emotional stress, toxins in your home and the environment around you can also contribute to illness, disease and aging. Poor choices do lead to problems.

Changing how you eat, think and live can help bring you back to homeostasis. You can start with the first step - eating an alkaline diet.

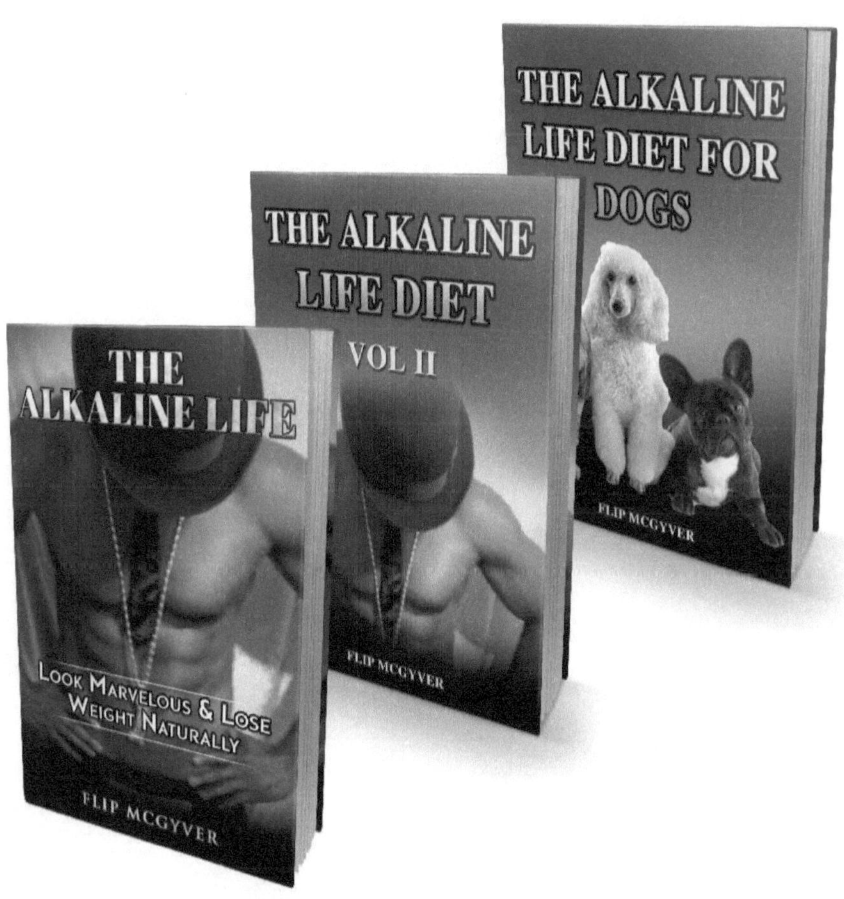

Thank you for allowing me to teach you about the benefits of having a ALKALINE body if you follow the steps outlined in this book you will better numerous aspects of your overall physical health to help you LIVE YOUR BEST LIFE…

Click here https://the-alkaline-life-diet.myshopify.com for more volumes in THE ALKALINE LIFE DIET SERIES

Thank you and good luck on your journey to a life of better health!